Prof. Arnold Ehret's

THE DEFINITE CURE OF CHRONIC CONSTIPATION

AND

OVERCOMING CONSTIPATION NATURALLY

Introduced & Edited by Prof. Spira

THE DEFINITE CURE OF CHRONIC CONSTIPATION

AND

OVERCOMING CONSTIPATION NATURALLY

By Prof. Arnold Ehret (1866-1922)

and Fred S. Hirsch

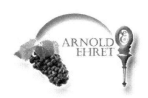

Copyright Breathair Publishing

Columbus, Ohio

2nd Edition 2014

Breathair Publishing
Columbus, Ohio

Available from www.mucusfreelife.com, Amazon.com, Kindle, and other retail outlets

Printed in the United States of America

Second Edition, 2014

ISBN-13: 978-0-99-065643-2
ISBN-10: 0-99-065643-8

www.mucusfreelife.com

Discover other titles by Breathair Publishing

Spira Speaks: Dialogs and Essays on the Mucusless Diet Healing System

Prof. Arnold Ehret's Rational Fasting for Physical, Mental and Spiritual Rejuvenation: Introduced and Edited by Prof. Spira

Thus Speaketh the Stomach and the Tragedy of Nutrition: Introduction by Prof. Spira

Coming Soon

Art of Transition: Spira's Mucusless Diet Healing System Menu and Recipe Guide

Table of Contents

Introduction

Professor Arnold Ehret was a German healer, dietitian, philosopher, teacher, visionary, and one of the first people to advocate fasting and a plant-based, vegan, mucus-free lifestyle as a therapy for healing. For over 100 years, his written works and teachings have touched the lives of thousands of health seekers pursuing higher levels of health. He was also a cultural icon who had a great influence on the "Back-to-Nature" counter-cultural movement which first emerged in Victorian Era Europe, and then migrated to Southern California in the early 1900s. The movement fundamentally influenced the hippie counter-culture of the 1960s.

In the early 1900s, Ehret opened a hugely popular sanitarium in Ascona, Switzerland where he treated and cured thousands of patients considered incurable by the so-called "medical authorities." During the latter part of the decade, Ehret engaged in a series of fasts monitored by German and Swiss officials. Within a period of 14 months, Ehret completed a fast of 21 days, one of 24 days, one of 32 days, and one of 49 days. He became one of the most in-demand health lecturers, journalists, and educators in Europe as he saved the lives of thousands of people.

On June 27, 1914, just before World War I, Ehret left from Bremen for the United States to see the Panama Exposition and sample the fruits of the continent. He found his way to California, which was viewed as an "Eden of the West." The region was also undergoing a horticultural renaissance due to botanists like Luther Burbank, which

3

greatly interested Ehret. The war prevented him from returning to Germany and he settled in Mount Washington, where he prepared his manuscripts and diplomas in his cultivated eating gardens. With the help of Fred Hirsch, he founded Ehret Literature and began to publish his masterful works.

Today, Ehret's works are increasing in popularity as people learn of the healing power of plant-based, vegan, and raw-food diets. Overall, Ehret believes that pus- and mucus-forming foods are unnatural for humans to eat. He asserts that a diet of fruits and green, leafy vegetables (i.e., mucus-free foods) are the most healing and powerful foods for humans. The world needs Ehret's work now more than ever. In an era where people consume genetically modified, mucus-forming *frankenfoods* daily, the simplicity and truthfulness of Ehret's teachings can transform humanity for the better.

In the *Definite Cure of Chronic Constipation and Overcoming Constipation Naturally*, Prof. Arnold Ehret and his number one student Fred Hirsch explore the generally constipated condition of the human organism. Such constipation is not only in the intestines, but also in the tissues and cells. This constipation is derived from unnatural, uneliminated accumulations of waste that build up in the human body from childhood on. Within, the authors explore how to fundamentally and DEFINITELY overcome the chronic constipation that plagues humanity. In this version, minor edits have been made to correct existing errors and outdated, gendered syntax.

-Prof. Spira

(2013)

4

The Definite Cure of Chronic Constipation

By Prof. Arnold Ehret

The Internal Uncleanliness of Man

Chronic constipation is the worst and most common crime against life and mankind—a crime unconsciously committed, and one whose full enormity is not yet fully realized. It stands accused of being one of the principal causative factors of all physical and mental diseases. I know as a fact, from my practical experience with thousands of chronically diseased, that the lives of humans, and the extent of their mental and spiritual capabilities, are largely influenced by the condition of the alimentary tract. It is certainly very important that the brain and nerves of men and women are supplied with pure blood, and are not dependent on blood polluted with impurities arising from an unclean alimentary canal. "Unclean" is too mild a word when we are dealing with the worst kind of a filthy condition.

It is a fact that humans, the product of the present "civilized" society of this much-vaunted "advanced" twentieth century, are born unhealthy because their mothers, during pregnancy, are almost invariably suffering from constipation. And I say further, that while in this state she usually eats two to three times as much as is necessary. This causes the so-called normal, more or less healthy person, to be somewhat encumbered from infancy. And to a much greater extent is the constipated one—who is loaded with such a mass of internal filth, that it can only be called "indescribable." His or her alimentary tract, reaching up from the mouth of the anus to his or her throat, is filled with a morbid mucus—undigested, decayed, and retained food substances, all of which are in a state of fermentation and putrefaction. Their intestines have never had a perfect cleansing during their entire life. At the conclusion of each discharge, the anus must be artificially cleansed, which shows that the internal walls of the intestines must also retain, after each passage, quantities of this same filth.

A physician of Berlin, whose lifework was the performing of autopsies, stated that 60 percent of all the corpses contained in the alimentary canal various foreign mater—worms and putrefied feces—and he further stated that in nearly all cases, the walls of the intestines and colon were lined with a crust of hardened feces, making it evident that these organs had degenerated to a state of utter inefficiency. Progressive American physicians are rapidly awakening to the fact that retained fecal matter is one of the chief causes of disease. Autopsies are constantly revealing indescribable, filthy, astounding conditions. One physician published the following:

> I have found a prototype of the cause of all diseases of the human body, the foundation of premature old age and death. Surprising as it may seem, out of 284 cases of autopsy held, but 28 colons were found to be free from hardened feces and in a normal and healthy state. The others, as described above, were to a more or less extent incrusted with hardened, rotten, rejected food material. Many were distended to twice their natural size throughout their whole length with a small hole through the center, and almost universally these last cases mentioned had regular bowel evacuations daily. Some of them contained large worms from four to six inches in length.
>
> My experience from day to day developed startling discoveries in the form of worms and nests of eggs, that we daily get from patients, accompanied by blood and pus. As I stood looking at the colon and reservoir of death, I expressed myself in wonder that anyone can live a week, much less for years, with such a cesspool of death and contagion always with him. The absorption of the deadly poison back into the circulation cannot help but cause all the contagious diseases. The recent treatment of hemorrhage of the bowels in typhoid fever has shown it to be caused by maggots and worms eating into the sensitive membrane and tapping a vein or artery. In fact, my experience during the past 10 years has proven, by the rapid recovery of all diseases after the colon was

cleansed, that in the colon itself lies the basic cause of almost all human ailments. —*Anonymous physician*

That this revolting and indescribable condition arises from the almost universal ignorance of right selection of food reveals why the *Mucusless Diet Healing System* is such an important discovery and development for the regeneration of humankind.

On the outside, the man or woman of today is carefully groomed, perhaps unnecessarily and over carefully clean; while inside, he or she is dirtier than the dirtiest animal—whose anus is as clean as its mouth, provided said animal has not been "domesticated" by "civilized" humans.

Long ago, naturopathy proved that in every disease there is a constitutional encumbrance of foreign matter, a clogging up of the system. That statement of fact is not sufficiently explicit. The encumbering matters, substances which would become dangerous if they were foreign to the body, and of no use to the system, consist of masses of accumulated feces, undigested food, morbid mucus, and retained superfluous water all in a state of fermentation and decomposition. Truly, chronically constipated people constantly carry in their intestines a veritable cesspool, by which the bloodstream is continually polluted and poisoned, a fact that only a skilled observer can at once detect by facial diagnosis. Official medical science and the inexpert layman do not suspect "constipation" when the individual consumes from three to five meals a day, while they are having one so-called, good bowel movement. Humans imagine that their "comfortably fatted" body is a sign of health; at the same time they are as much in fear of a cold wind and "germs" as they are of the devil. When such a "well-fed" person who is usually constipated takes a fast or is put on a "mucusless diet"—as I have advised hundreds as their last resort—will discharge masses of putrescent filth, fetid urine loaded with mucus, salt, uric acid, fat, drugs, albumen and pus, all according to their diseases.

The most surprising effect of these treatments is the immense quantity of the discharged feces and the fetid exhalation from both the mouth and skin. But the most important "discharge" is the elimination through the circulation into the urine. The urine of everybody will then show sediment of mucus as soon as he or she fasts a little or reduces the quantity of food, or makes a change toward natural, mucus-free foods. Doctors call it "disease," and it is in fact a self-cleansing process of the body.

This self-elimination through the circulation is the body's most wonderful healing work of every disease. To control this process by food and food quantities is the only true, natural, and most perfect therapeutic art of healing, and is in no other "treatment" so successfully accomplished as in the *Mucusless Diet Healing System*.

This elimination—especially that of the sick person after a long period of misery, suffering, and unsuccessful medical treatment—is human's "greatest event." He or she now realizes what they have never thought of—and what only a few physicians in the world have ever understood as I did, through thousands of cases—that mostly all civilized people are walking, living cesspools, due to chronic constipation.

All of his or her former unsuccessful treatments now appear to them in a tragic-comical light. They now know exactly where the source of their suffering is to be found, no matter what the name of the disease may be. They now understand that they were wrongly and ignorantly treated by the doctors who "suppressed the disease" without eliminating the filth that was retained in their entire system, especially in his or her alimentary canal, since childhood, and which condition constituted the principal causative factor of the disease.

The Effect of Laxatives

I believe that neither physicians nor laypersons really know or understand how and why the body performs the laxative effect of these different remedies. Official medical science knows very little about the "why" of the drugs. Their application is based upon the experience only that each one has "a special effect."

All laxatives contain more or less poisons, that is, to enter the circulation in a concentrated form. The protective instinct of the body reacts instantly by a greater water supply into the stomach from the blood in order to dissolve and weaken the dangerous substance; the intestines are stimulated for increased and quickened activity, and so the "solution" is discharged, only taking parts of the feces along. This is the physiological explanation, and you can see that the effect is an abnormal stimulation of vitality in general and of the intestinal

8

nerves in particular. It is an open secret that all laxatives finally fail, because the constantly overloaded intestines are being overstimulated by the laxatives and thereby slowly paralyzed. To continually increase the laxatives year after year, instead of changing the diet, means SUICIDE—slow, but sure.

The Real and Deeper Cause of Constipation

Constipation itself is a disease, and a really "severe" one, at that, because in severe cases it burdens the system with a heavy load of filth, sometimes weighing as much as 10 pounds or more. Disease as such is an abnormal, unnatural condition; even "orthodox" physicians agree on that. We should expire slowly and painlessly, when vitality is exhausted, had we not lived with disease and suffering. That cases of "natural death" are becoming more infrequent nowadays, which is further proof of the depths we have sunken into in the "swamps of civilization."

Constipation—this most common disease—has not decreased or improved in spite of thousands of remedies for sale on the market, and in spite of so-called medical science; simply, because the "diet of civilization" is unnatural. The human intestines are not organized at all for this unnatural food either to digest it perfectly or to expel the unused residue.

Very little is known about foods that are constipating and those of the opposite kind. What I wrote and proved in my book *Rational Fasting and Regeneration Diet* regarding the fundamental causative factors of all diseases constitutes the deepest insight known into the nature of chronic constipation.

Don't you know that bookbinder's paste is made of fine white flour, rice, or potatoes? That glue is made from flesh, gristle, and bones? Don't you know how sticky these substances are? Don't you know that skimmed milk, buttermilk, and cream are the best ingredients to furnish sticky base for colors for painting? That the white of eggs will stick paper or cloths so perfectly that it resists dissolution in water? Every housewife and cook knows how oils and fats stick to the sides of a pan. At least 90 percent of the "diet of civilization" contains these sticky foods, and humans stuff themselves daily with awful mixtures of them. Thus, the digestive tract is not only clogged up through constipation but literally glued together with sticky mucus and feces.

Herewith, the "mystery" of chronic constipation is unveiled and the story told of the fundamental causative factor of all diseases. Disease is but internal uncleanliness—this simply states a true but woeful fact. Fruits, green-leaf and starchless vegetables do not contain these pasty, gluey mucus substances and are natural foods—yet little credit has been given them by doctors or laypersons. I will lift the veil and show why they fail to understand. Fruit acids and mineral-rich vegetable juices dissolve the pasty mucus encumbrances. Fruit sugar causes and develops their fermentation and forms gases. This so greatly feared fermentation of the inside filth is another necessary stirring up "process" to prepare them for elimination. Acid and fermented starch and glue lose their sticky ability as soon as they ferment. If an average meat eater or a child fed mostly on starchy foods accidentally eats too freely of good, sweet fruits, a "revolution" in the alimentary canal with diarrhea usually sets in, and fever is caused through the increased fermentation.

In severe cases, if a doctor stops the diarrhea and feeds, as is usually the procedure, the patient dies, because Nature was kept from accomplishing the cleansing process. The partly dissolved poisons remain in the system, causing death.

The patient literally suffocates in their own mire of filth, accumulated during their life from wrong food material and overeating. If the patient does not die, their case ordinarily becomes chronic, which means Nature is continually trying to expel poisonous mucus and gases in spite of all obstructions and counteracting remedies. The constipation merely aggravates the process. Instead of eating less and then only loosening foods, the chronic patient stuffs himself more and more with wrong foods, becomes fatter every day, and even takes pleasure in their increased weight. In fact, this overweight, called health by the misguided ones, is mostly accumulated feces—water—and various kinds of filth. In most cases of tuberculosis, these conditions are typical. Five to six meals a day and one bowel movement or even less—no wonder he takes on weight, looks "full of vigor"—but can never be cured.

Nourishing and Curing Laxatives

No advance physician will deny the relation between any disease and constipation. But today people are far away from Nature and the truth, and they are kept more and more in darkness—when taken sick, they do just the opposite of what they should do. The slightest indisposition, a little headache or cold, which is the result of insufficient bowel movement, is treated with more and so-called better eating—in spite of a decreased appetite. This is the main reason why influenza, the "flu," became a fatal disease. Formerly "flu" was as easy to cure as the harmless "Grippe"—a self-cleansing process of the body, mostly prevalent in springtime. Knowing nothing of "scientific medicine," germs, etc., the patient instinctively followed their lack of appetite, took a mild laxative, and very rapidly recovered; usually they felt much better after than before the "healing" disease. Today, he or she is falsely taught that a germ is responsible—and not his or her dangerous unhygienic habits. They eat too much, which is against the law of Nature, instead of fasting the way every ailing animal cures itself. But the amount of internal impurities and autotoxins of humans exceed those of any diseased animal. A long fast, therefore, would kill the majority of sick people; however, they would not die by starvation, but would become suffocated from their own poisonous filth. As an authority in fasting, I know full well the reason why a fast is so feared by most people, and that it has been misapplied by laypersons. It is a crime to advise a constipated patient to fast until their tongue is clean before removing the "deposits of poisons" from his or her intestines. I could only succeed in curing very old, severe cases of chronic constipation by relatively long fasts. Humans, in regard to health, are more degenerated than any kind of animal. Men and women have lost their reason, so to say, about matters of which they think the animal has none at all. Yet, their intelligence places them far above the animal and enables them to assist Nature to overcome obstructions and difficulties that could become dangerous. That is the philosophical sense of the Art of Naturopathy.

Therefore, if you want to cure chronic constipation perfectly and without any harm, you must change your diet, and instead of using foods that produce disease and constipation eat really nourishing foods which loosen up, dissolve, and cure. But people are ignorant

11

regarding this truth, just as they are about fasting, and they try to do things without previous experience or knowledge, and failure is usually the result. What I call mucusless diet consists of fresh, ripe fruits and starchless vegetables, for they are the ideal foods and the fundamental remedies for all diseases. Of course, the application must be intelligently advised by a practitioner graduated from my school of the *Mucusless Diet Healing System*, or a personal knowledge can be received through the study of my book, the *Mucusless Diet Healing System*.

It is an "eating-your-way-to-health" treatment and consequently, the most reasonable method of curing, because wrong eating is the causative factor in all diseases.

These mucusless, nourishing, and "laxative" (that is, dissolving) foods form new blood; the best blood that has ever run through your veins—and at once start the so-called constitutional cure of the body. The circulation of the new blood, permeating every part of the system, dissolves and eliminates the morbid mucus, which is clogging up the entire human organism; it especially loosens the deep-seated impurities in the intestines and renovates the whole system. This then, is the great enlightening fact—why constipation not only can be perfectly cured but why the mucusless diet cures when all other treatments have failed.

In severe cases of chronic constipation, it is advisable in the beginning to use as a help a harmless laxative to remove the solid obstructions of feces in the intestines; in other words, to eject the worst filth out of a clogged-up pipe system. Enemas consisting of clear, warm water are also a good help in the beginning.

Among numerous laxatives on the market, those of botanical origin are the least harmful. After many years of experience, I have prepared a "special mixture" of this kind. It has the advantage of removing the old, solid feces, obstructions, and mucus from the intestines without causing the usual diarrhea and constipation as an aftereffect. It is to be used in the beginning only, as an aid, and will not have to be used continually. As soon as the intestines are cleansed from the retained masses of feces and other obstructions, and the mucusless or mucus-lean diet is taken up, you will realize the truth of the previously stated facts. You will then perceive with both your eyes and with your nose

12

that I have not exaggerated. And you will become convinced that the state of obstruction was not only localized in your intestines but that all passages of your entire system were obstructed and constipated with mucus from your head to your toes.

You will then experience the formerly unbelievable fact that any kind of disease—even those considered incurable by all doctors—under my treatment soon begins to improve and is finally cured, if a cure is at all possible, simply because the source of poisoning of the system—the chronic constipation—is eliminated. Then the new blood, derived from natural food, circulates "unpoisoned" through the entire system and dissolves and eliminates every local symptom, even in the most deep-seated cases; and it removes the impurities of the entire system, which were mainly supplied from the deposits of poisons and morbid mucus in the intestines, which condition is called Chronic Constipation.

Conclusion

"Life is a tragedy of nutrition" is a statement I made many years ago. Everyone knows we dig our graves with our teeth, but the saddest of all is the present-day superstition of 995 of the people—the most highly educated and the ignorant—the healthy as well as sick—the rich and the poor—that we must eat more concentrated food when weak or sick. Concentrated food, high protein and starchy foods, are the most constipating, which, as shown in this booklet, accumulate in the form of waste in the alimentary canal. The so-called "good stool" daily is in reality constipation, and you may now see that constipation is the main source of every disease and that the average person suffering from constipation can only be healed perfectly by a diet, free from STICKY—GLUEY—PASTY properties and that is a MUCUSLESS DIET.

You may improve your elimination temporarily through laxative remedies—special physical exercises—vibration, massages, and various other methods, but you cannot clean out the old obstructions from the alimentary canal and regenerate and cleanse the whole system as long as you eat the same mucus- and toxic-forming foods which have caused, and continue causing, your constipation and all other ailments of the human body.

Overcoming Constipation Naturally

By Fred S. Hirsch

Neither time nor money has been spared by the best talents known to the medical profession in an attempt to unravel the mystery of constipation, its causes, and cure. No drug has as yet been compounded capable of permanently overcoming intestinal stasis. The problem of constipation remains a "problem" after thousands of years!

Arnold Ehret, in his book *Mucusless Diet Healing System*, describes it thusly: "Constipation results from a congestion of a capillary circulation brought about through excessive mucus and impurities (foreign waste matter) clogging up the bloodstream and tissue system, to the external circulation that is impeded, causing inability to discharge the natural flow of fecal matter normally." In other words, loss of proper peristaltic movement of the intestines causes failure of the bowels to evacuate the unwanted waste fecal matter normally.

It would almost appear repetitive to further describe just what constipation is—or how in so many different ways it can harmfully affect the human body; but only through constant reiteration will full enlightenment bring the necessary knowledge of this most important subject. The various painful afflictions resulting from constipation have been given many "scientific names" descriptive of the actual organ or particular part of the body affected. Constipation is a blocking-up of the human "sewage system" and makes of humans a "walking

15

cesspool!" Can you think of anything more repulsive than forced retention within the body of putrid, decaying, germ-laden, "sewage"? Would you willingly reside beside an open cesspool? Most certainly NOT! And yet this is exactly what the constipated individual is doing. We use perfumed soaps to counteract body odors and resort to a "mouthwash" to "kill" bad breath. Just so long as the type of food you eat starts decaying and putrefying if allowed to remain impacted between the teeth, then "brushing your teeth after every meal" is a must. It seems unbelievable that we persist in eating these very foods in the unmistakably false belief that they are essential to life! What further proof is needed that they are the direct cause of our ailments?

Within this wonderful body of ours is contained a natural, miraculous ability to overcome intestinal sluggishness and the many other various ailments to which humans are prey. All that is necessary on your part is to provide the proper kind of food Nature demands to restore normal bowel activity. The method of correction is extremely simple, but neglect through ignorance or otherwise to heed Nature's warning will eventually result in a complete "breakdown." There can be no compromise; you have violated Nature's law and a plea of innocent is unacceptable; you must now pay the penalty. Either prompt removal of all "surplus garbage" or else! The bowels are overloaded, and this "blockage" cannot be tolerated. The necessary vitality needed to carry on, is lacking.

A complete cessation of the causes is the only possible hope. Stimulating bowel action through use of violent purgatives is equal to attempting to spur on an already exhausted horse to further effort! Only through complete cooperation can you hope for a "pardon." What a surprising "relief" results in your physical condition through following this rational health regime.

The One-ness of Disease
There is only one disease, although its manifestations are various, and there is but one cause, and that is retention of waste matters. Bias, prejudice, and erratic conclusions have always stood in the way of progress!

Presumably, you are in earnest and desire to attain virile, vital, normal, *good* health—otherwise you would not be reading this article. Good health requires dedication of purpose and unwavering observance of all Health rules. "Wishful thinking" must be replaced with "positive thinking"; halfway measures bring only halfway results. The power to heal is invested in the individual. We must therefore do our own curing! Is gluttony your supreme source to pleasure in life, and if so, are you willing to exchange it for other, more worthwhile enjoyments? Your acquired "taste buds" will soon be replaced with natural desires and you will soon find yourself enjoying pleasure in eating as formerly. Social activities might change, but new friends will be found to take the place of those who might misunderstand. Your desire to remain young, energetic, and vivaciously healthy must prevail. When this takes place, vital forces are restored to a normal balance and mental and physical alertness returns. Every mouthful of Natural food is delicious to the taste, and life takes on an entirely new meaning of joyful activity.

Physical Exercises Are Necessary

Strengthening your flaccid abdominal muscles is most important, since proper bowel function requires strong abdominal muscular ability. Use of the "slanting board" is particularly helpful in building abdominal muscular strength without overtaxing your strength. Lie flat on your back and with hands clasped behind the head, try to bring the body to a sitting position. You may at first find it necessary to have your legs and feet held down until the abdominal muscles become stronger. Walking is one of the very best exercises and a daily walk of not less than 15 minutes should become a MUST, for walking opens up new avenues of blood circulation in dormant areas. You can easily combine breathing exercises with walking. Inhale sharply through the nose on four counts—then hold the breath four counts; now exhale completely for four counts, and again hold the breath four counts—then start all over again. Use pure sparkling water if available—otherwise distilled water with the addition of a few drops of fresh lemon juice to replace the minerals lost by distillation. You may drink as much as you desire between meals, but no liquids with meals. We must learn how to restore lost health in order to retain good health indefinitely.

White Blood Corpuscle and Anemic Paleness

Humans today are pathologically sick. The anemic paleness and pallid white skin are visual indications that all is not well! Health authorities agree that serious recognition must be given the matter of complete and thorough bowel elimination. Ehret states in his book the

Mucusless Diet Healing System, "Overeating of starchy foods such as wheat and grain products, breads, cakes, pastries, and pies, and the dairy products: butter, cheese, eggs, and pasteurized milk (i.e., acid-forming foods) tend to produce an excess of white blood corpuscles, mucus, and similar waste encumbrances, all of which directly and indirectly contribute to chronic constipation. To restore a ruddy, natural skin color with its vibrant healthy glow; the 'red corpuscles' must predominate."

Keep the Colon Clean

How often have you delayed answering Nature's first call because you were "too busy," or the time was "inopportune," and many other reasons? "Housebroken" pets become constipated from this same "delaying habit." Don't fail to answer Nature's call immediately upon the very first warning! Retention or delay for too long a period can result in reabsorption of the semi-liquid poisonous wastes in the intestines directly into the circulation through the bloodstream; the remaining feces becomes dry, elimination is more difficult, and an impaction of the bowels results. The simple headache, nervous tensions, muscular aches and pains, dizziness, lack of vitality, and many of the common types of ailments are directly traceable to constipation. Cellular degeneration causing serious ailments eventually follow, and unless we can re-establish healthy, natural bowel movements through a thorough cleansing, disease becomes rampant. Here, in a nutshell, lies the secret of disease.

With a clogged bowel system, illness is bound to be present. Despite the repeated medical assurance that "aspirin type" remedies are harmless, we are bluntly informed by the manufacturer that "relief" is "temporary" at best. Yes, indeed, it will require a lot of COURAGE, PATIENCE, PERSEVERANCE, AND FAITH on your part— before the elusive Fountain of Youth is attained.

Maintain a Normal Bowel Functioning

Prof. Arnold Ehret in his *Mucusless Diet Healing System* claimed CONSTIPATION to be the primary cause of 99.9 percent of all human ills, including the so-called "incurable diseases," i.e., cancer, tuberculosis, diabetes, arthritis, tumors, and many others; in fact, practically every ailment to which the human body is prey! Dr. J. H. Kellogg of Battle Creek Sanitarium shares this opinion, for he stated,

18

"ALL CANCER PATIENTS ARE VICTIMS OF CHRONIC CONSTIPATION!"

We herewith submit a "suggestion" primarily intended for our male readers only, since women have followed this practice for thousands of years! The "suggestion" has proven to be exceptionally effective in aiding and correcting normal bowel functioning! Could it be that this is the answer to the age-old question, "Why do women enjoy greater longevity than men, normally outliving their male companions of many years?"

It seems that both men and women find ready excuses for postponing "Nature's call," failing to recognize the seriousness of the occasion! Please—for your health's sake and beginning with RIGHT NOW!—promise yourself never to delay answering "Nature's call" IMMEDIATELY! It can prove to be tremendously important to your future good health and well-being! To postpone this important function is a direct cause of resulting constipation, which eventually becomes "chronic." Strange, isn't it, that when hunger "calls" we readily find time to stop and eat!

The advice offered to our "male" readers is extremely simple and easy to follow! Instead of your continuing the present, "time-saving" custom of "standing" upright while urinating, we recommend "sitting" on the toilet bowl—in a squatting position and at the same time concentrating on having a bowel movement! This may mean a few minutes extra time—but it will surely prove time well spent in improving your health! Patience is required, and possibly 10 or more minutes may be necessary during the "habit-forming" period. It won't be long though, in fact, 1 or 2 weeks should find you happily experiencing "normal" bowel movements! We are all "creatures of habit," and this "good habit" is surely definitely worth cultivating! For nothing can be of greater importance to all of us than GOOD HEALTH! "When you have your health, you have everything!"

These suggestions are equally important for women who consider themselves too busy to spare the extra few minutes required. Yet, they spend weeks or months recovering from a costly surgical operation. Decide RIGHT NOW to follow these simple suggestions—you won't regret it! Start TODAY, not TOMORROW, and make it a daily MUST, every day, for the remainder of your life!

19

Remember, "Mother Nature" accepts NO EXCUSES! She desires ALL of her beloved "children" to be healthy. Are you aware that we normally should experience a bowel movement within not more than 3 hours after each meal! THIS COULD BE THE SECRET OF GOOD HEALTH!

The ancient Greeks made a practice of "sleeping-off" all types of illness. Their hospitals were known as "Temples of Sleep" and the patient was kept sleeping during the entire convalescent period. Actually what took place was that the body was undergoing the "fasting cure" and the digestive organs received a much needed rest. Our hardworking kidneys, liver, stomach, in fact the entire intestinal tract require this occasional rest, just as do the involuntary muscles of the body. Under normal conditions, Nature takes care of this "rest period" during a sound undisturbed sleep. Going without food for a few days provides a physiological rest required by our digestive organs. Here's an easy experiment well worth trying: Upon arising, drink a full glass of hot water to which the juice of one-half fresh lemon has been added and honey may be added to taste. For your noon meal the next 3 or 4 days, eat only an apple with dried figs. Nothing else! The evening meal can consist of a green-leaf salad, grated carrots, and sliced celery. Such a series of short fasts of 2 or 3 days each, if followed over a period of 2 or 3 months, will prove most beneficial. Your sleep will be restful, you will awaken in the morning with zest; more vitality will be noted, and your mental attitude toward the rest of the world might even improve! Eliminating "waste materials" is just as essential as sufficient food intake.

The Habit of Overeating
Overcoming a lifelong habit of "overeating" is a difficult problem for the habitually constipated; "habit" is the motivating desire to eat rather than normal hunger. The average 'food eater' often consumes as much as five times more food than necessary. Valuable energy is *needlessly wasted digesting* the surplus food, which remains in the intestines in an undigested mass of decaying, decomposing "garbage." Nature's method of saving the individual's life from self-poisoning is to "store" this surplus waste in the tissue system awaiting more opportune time to dispose of same! These poisonous wastes are re-absorbed over and over again, polluting the bloodstream. The source of supply of these disease-breeding wastes must be stopped. Every

effort to remedy the condition must be initiated, aiding nature to cleanse the tissues and help bring about a normal, healthy condition of regularity.

The use of chemical fertilizers and poisonous sprays have come into popularity because of their ability to increase crop yield. But sad to say, it has been proven that fruits and vegetables grown in chemically treated soil lack the proper vital mineral contents and they can also create an additional health hazard. Be as selective as possible when buying your vegetables at supermarkets, and when possible, select those grown in organically treated soils. Many modern health food stores now supply organically grown fruits and vegetables that meet these requirements.

Who Are the Constipated?
"Constipation is one of the most frequent conditions that the physician is called upon to treat, yet there is probably no other common disorder which occurs so often and is so badly managed," observed Dr. H. L. Cockus, MD in *Gastroenterogy Vol. 11*. Dr. Jerome Marks, MD writes in *Dietetics for the Clinician*, "Constipation exists when an individual does not spontaneously evacuate the bowel at least once in 24 hours." This condition—also called "intestinal sluggishness"—is the result of wrong living according to Dr. Robert G. Jackson. MD, and we find in his book *How to be Always Well* that "the bacteria of putrefaction multiply with numerous rapidity." They not only produce poisons that pass into the blood and burden the organs of elimination, but they locally irritate and could set up an inflammatory state in the lining of the bowel, known to the physician as colitis. Constipation may seem a simple thing, but its proper treatment is a matter of great importance to the well-being of the individual. Ultimate success requires close cooperation.

A gradual process of elimination, depending entirely on the individual's physical condition, is the proper procedure. Avoid trying to "rush" nature, for it may become dangerous to stir up the "poisonous wastes" too rapidly!

Survival of our Present Civilization

We are not attempting to predict the end of civilization in claiming that if humans are to survive, they must soon make a decision between returning to natural foods or continuing on today's accepted diet of demineralized and devitalized "foodless foods" with its certainty of sickness, painful ailments, and a shortened life. All you need do is read the labels on any food package! The manufacturer adds certain preservatives to make their food product a good "shelf item" (i.e., one with "long-keeping" qualities). Artificial coloring and artificial sweetener make the item more appetizing, and the chemical additives are used for various purposes, many of which are trade secrets known only to the manufacturer. Through a recent discovery, a chemical spray has been perfected making it possible to keep vegetables such as lettuce and other greens as crisp and fresh for weeks—as when first harvested! The time is rapidly approaching; if our present civilization is to survive, we must *take action*, we owe it to the unborn generation who will follow us! The poisonous chemicals used for "crop dusting" and for spraying trees have succeeded in not only destroying the unfriendly insects but friendly ones as well! Our "good earth" contains many friendly earthworms and friendly bacteria intended by Nature to fertilize and purify the soil, and they have become innocent victims of chemical poisoning! We are rapidly reaching the point where the soil can no longer supply the fruits and vegetables with the necessary minerals and vitamins required for our very existence! How much longer can life continue! Or perhaps, a better question would be, "How much longer will we allow this to continue?"

Many books on this subject have been written sounding their note of warning and are readily available at any public library, but they go practically unheeded. It is too much to hope that sooner or later, through increased experience, our health authorities will accept this knowledge, which is the only salvation for abundant healthful life.

Physical Suffering and Mental Unrest

More illness, nervous breakdowns, and suffering from mental unrest has been caused through eating wrong foods than through any other source. It is fairly safe to say that the average person eats what they like, when they like, and as much as they like without giving too much consideration to what the end results might be. So in searching for the probable cause of physical or mental breakdown, even in individuals who have lived more or less faultless lives "dietetically speaking," we still find food to be the chief offender! It is, of course, essential that the individual recognize this fact and is self-convinced and willingly corrects his or her dietetic shortcomings. While stressing the importance of food, we must not overlook other important factors such as the need of a happy mental attitude, nor sufficient sleep, nor healthy working habits. Sickness is much less likely to obtain a foothold when all of these facts are given their due consideration. Modern food preservatives and chemical additives were unknown when Grandma was a child and "gout" was a sign of wealth! It is unreasonable to assume that we prepare our meals of today just as mankind has existed on for thousands of years past! The Bible mentions the longevity of biblical characters. The present-day art of food preparation is a recent discovery. Our ancestors' foods were much simpler. With the coming of more densely populated towns, disease became rampant, and they learned the "hard way" the lesson that "cleanliness is next to Godliness." After the European and Middle East plagues that threatened to destroy all humankind, the very streets were scrubbed immaculately clean. Modern sanitation, filtered water, sanitary plumbing, and public sewerage systems are presently a must in Western civilization, but we still fail to recognize the essential necessity of "internal cleanliness" for humans themselves; and the average individual carries around as much as 10 pounds of uneliminated fecal matter in his or her body, falsely considering this extra poundage as being "healthy." Our government Food & Drug authorities are graduates of the same colleges as the scientists in the employ of the large commercial chemical concerns who, through research and development in their respective laboratories, concoct the chemical food additives. The government maintains at considerable public expense large testing laboratories of their own, and while admittedly acknowledging that artificial coloring, chemically produced sweetening, and similar food additives are known to be harmful in large dosage and have been proven to produce many ailments, they are permissible—"acceptable" because only small portions are used in the food product and are therefore supposedly harmless.

We have more than sufficient and ample proof of the constipating effects of human-made "foodless foods," yet hardly a day goes by but what some highly ranked scientist issues a startling announcement of having perfected a "patented" chemical concoction capable of supplying the required food concentrate sufficient to feed the entire present population of the world at practically no cost whatsoever! While possibly on the same date, another equally well known scientist warns that over 50 percent of the "underprivileged" in the United States are dying from "malnutrition!" The actual truth is the individual can no longer find proper nourishment in the foods they must now accept! Urging the discontinuance of poisonous sprays and chemical fertilizers is in the interest of food preservation! Try to imagine, if you can, the tremendous quantity of poisonous pollutants. Millions of tons of poison dusts released daily by planes, automobiles, motor trucks, oil refineries, steel mills, and factories belching forth poisonous waste gases and other poisons into the air we are forced to breathe! The health of every individual, man, woman, and child is threatened. Every living creature, both on land and sea—yes, every living plant—all are faced with eventual extinction unless this most serious situation is corrected—and soon! Scientists report that an analysis of the purest snow known to humans—taken at the extreme point of the South Pole—contain traces of "atomic fallout." Contamination of our water and air must not be tolerated at any cost! What percentage of the causes of constipation can be blamed on the chlorine and other chemicals now being added to the water supplies of our large metropolitan areas? And the dental profession has joined the ranks, favoring compulsory "fluoridation" of our drinking water on the basis of "fewer cavities" for the children! These chemicals are so destructive that they require "special containers," since chlorine can eat through a steel tank!

Mental Unrest

Constipation, when caused through "overeating" and improper food preparation, is a prime contributor to the condition known as "mental unrest" and "nervous breakdowns." Our health authorities are aware of these facts and recognize that the human nervous system is poisoned by impurities from the waste products of constipation that enter the bloodstream. Nature has provided many "safety devices" to insure that only the "purest" blood feeds the brain cells—but often Nature is unable to cope with the situation. Impurities in the blood supply to the brain make normal functioning of that most important organ inefficient and befuddled. Prof. Ehret, in his writings, tells of many mental cases that came under his observation. Most of them responded favorably to fasting and proper diet! The "mental patient," in a majority of cases, has eaten foods especially rich in "protein" for many years previous to their "breakdown." With the total discontinuance of protein foods such as meat, eggs, milk, and cheese, excellent results were obtained! Even some mental cases caused through physical injuries or sudden shock—uncontrollable grief or severe fright—have been known to respond to a fruitarian and starch-free diet.

Medical Examinations

The value of medical examinations is not to be underestimated—but in a majority of cases, *results* and not *cause* are given most consideration by the examining physician. Nature has provided a self-diagnosis, which Ehret named the "Magic Mirror." Expensive laboratory equipment is unnecessary to safely diagnose your latent disease. The coated tongue, foul breath, clouded urine, putrid fecal matter, puffiness under the eyes, excessive release of phlegm (mucus) through the nose, and expectoration, swollen ankles, offensive odors from both under arm and feet, inflamed eyes—to mention but a few—are visible signs that herald in advance your failing physical condition. Perhaps you are one of the thousands of well-meaning individuals who have dutifully undergone a series of physical tests, spent your good time and money for a "complete physical," and upon receiving the doctor's report and being told that a corrective diet was essentially necessary, you "attempted"—although rather feebly—to do your part and follow the doctor's good advice; but through lack of "willpower," "faulty" eating habits were resumed and you were soon back "enjoying poor health." Very often, unfortunately, full realization comes too late! Hopefully, you still have time, for "where there is life, there is hope." But Nature must be given the opportunity and you must cooperate!

Longevity Obtainable

Humans have undoubtedly shortened their normal span of life through excessive food intake and improper living habits. Modern sanitation corrected past scourges of pestilence such as typhoid, cholera, bubonic plague, yellow fever, and scarlet fever. Hundreds of thousands of lives were lost and entire cities wiped out, yet humans permit the contamination of their precious life-giving "bloodstream" to continue unheeded! Medical practitioners now accept the possibility of human's life expectancy increasing to as much as 200 years! While their claims are based primarily on the efficacy of modern surgery (i.e., transplantation of vital organs), the willingness on their part to admit that the human machine is capable of continuing for this added length of time is quite a concession. Drugless practitioners, on the other hand, based longevity through a return to simplicity in our eating habits—especially the avoidance of overeating. All doctors agree that the majority overeat as much as five times more food than the body requires. Based on this presumption; we use five times more "vitality" than we normally should in disposing of food surplus. The Hunza people are a living example of what "simple," natural living will do for longevity! Women who have reached the age of 150 years give birth to children sired by husbands the same age and even older!

One suggested method of reducing food consumption is to follow a non-breakfast plan. We have health advocates recommending the first meal at 10:00 a.m. and the next at 4:30 or 5:00 p.m. Prof. Ehret—a 'two-meal-per-day plan' advocate—suggested the first meal be at noon and the evening meal at 6:00 p.m. Here is the plan I have been following over the past 50 years: Upon arising, a full glass of hot water to which the juice of half a lemon and pure honey to taste has been added. This helps cleanse the alimentary canal. Many ardent health disciples follow a "one-meal-a-day plan' eaten at about 4:30 p.m.; it practically means a daily fast! No solid foods are taken, although pure water or fruit juices are permissible. Whatever plan you follow, you will notice that the reduction in quantity of food intake will bring about a gradual improvement in your health, and constipation disappears! The sufferer from chronic constipation must seek permanent relief through their choice of foods from the vegetable kingdom, i.e., fruits and green-leaf, starchless vegetables, since they have no other alternative! All vegetables are rich in valuable mineral content, i.e., iron, calcium, sodium, magnesium, carbohydrates, vitamins, and especially Vitamins A, B, and C. Fresh fruits and starchless vegetables are alkaline, or "mucusless," whereas grains and cereals are "acid-forming" and definitely "mucus-forming." Dairy products come under the classification of "acid-forming." When preparing edible "starchy" vegetables, it is suggested that they be

26

thoroughly baked, making them more easily digested. Coleslaw is prepared by slicing the cabbage finely, then adding lemon juice and a little olive oil (cabbage is often gas-forming, and the lemon juice lessens this tendency). Add chopped celery to the mix. You will find it to be tasty and an excellent "cleanser." If desired, a little salt may be added. Cooked spinach, beet tops, and baked beets can be added. This makes a most satisfying meal, which will also prove "laxative." You will find many similar Ehret recipes in his *Mucusless Diet* Lesson Course.

Basic Rules for a Disease-Free, Healthy Life

Constipation need no longer be a "mystery," for you have now been informed of all the measures necessary to overcome the most stubborn cases. Recognition of internal uncleanliness as disease producing should make you desirous of overcoming your constipation, and the few following rules are submitted for further consideration. Distress that frequently follows eating is unfortunately too well known! The pathological effects are not thoroughly understood at present by the great majority.

1. TO LENGTHEN YOUR LIFE, SHORTEN YOUR MEALS! Eat slowly and relish your food, for food must be appetizing and thoroughly masticated in order to digest properly. The first stage of digestion takes place in the mouth; hence the necessity of thorough mastication. To avoid overeating, it is a good rule to leave the table while still hungry! Avoid eating between meals!

2. Avoid drinking any liquids with meals. This includes water, tea, milk, coffee, fruit juices, and even soups. Wait at least 15 minutes after drinking before you start eating solid foods. And wait at least the same length of time after eating solids before you drink liquids. Liquids interfere with digestion of your food when taken together.

3. Avoid all harsh condiments and spices. This includes salt, pepper, mustard, ketchup, vinegar, pickles, etc. They may stimulate jaded appetites but digestion is retarded.

4. Avoid using butter, margarine, and most cooking oils. Use pure olive oil where necessary to prevent sticking to baking dish. Starchy vegetables should be steamed or boiled until soft enough to insert fork easily, then baked for at least 30 minutes or

until thoroughly dextrinized. You will find added flavor through baking, and also the food becomes more easily digestible.

5. Avoid all denatured and overprocessed foods such as white flour and "ready to use" cake mixes. Prepared "TV" frozen dinners should also be avoided. All nourishing content has been dissipated through the processor's use to food preservatives and chemical additives. A more nutritional meal would consist of a salad of fresh greens, cottage cheese, tomatoes, and one or two cooked vegetables. Or better still, a fruit salad with yogurt or cottage cheese. Dried figs, dates, apricots, or raisins chewed together with a few nuts until thoroughly masticated furnish the necessary protein the body requires. Avocadoes also have high protein content and are rich in poly-unsaturated fat, but eat sparingly.

6. Avoid constipating foods such as mashed potatoes with gravy, hot buns, cakes, and pastries and cooked cereals of all kinds. Dairy products—eggs, milk, cheese, and butter—are constipating and form toxic-waste poisons in the body and should be avoided.

7. Avoid all frozen desserts such as ice creams, sherbets, etc. Frozen desserts "shock" the digestive apparatus, and have a high acid content. They rob the system of valuable Vitality. The too liberal use of eggs and milk can cause putrefaction in the digestive track; normal functioning is impeded and poisons that should have been eliminated are retained.

8. Since humans are "creatures of habit," it is wise to take advantage of this fact. Make it a daily "habit" to visit the bathroom the very first thing in the morning or immediately after eating. Allow yourself ample time; concentrate on elimination taking place. Be willing to spend 15 or 20 minutes if necessary— during the "experimental stage." It may require some time before Nature accepts the suggestion! You may use bulb syringe—with lukewarm, not hot, water when necessary, retaining *the water at least 10 minutes before rejecting.* You will eventually be rewarded with

permanent regularity, particularly if a corrective diet, proper physical exercises, and deep breathing has been followed.[1]

The Cleansing Diet

Constipation is a direct invitation to disease! Constipation causes a depletion in energy, and Prof. Ehret makes this clear in his book *Mucusless Diet Healing System* in Lesson 5. Ehret's explanation of how vital energy becomes lost through excessive "obstruction" is understandable. "Weight is disease," he states, "and you will lose weight at first through following a natural food diet, especially through use of fruit juices recommended on the 'cleansing diet'— but this 'weight' consisting of 'waste encumbrances' is the direct cause of your illness and misery." There are many excellent, moderately priced juicing machines now available for making vegetable juices at home. Apple or prune juice can be purchased at all supermarkets. Fresh orange and grapefruit juice are easily made at home. Certain juices will be found more laxative than others. Prune juice is always available and is an excellent "laxative." Fresh coconut juice ,when mixed with fresh (not canned) carrot juice, makes a delicious tasty drink with laxative qualities. Both fresh orange and grapefruit juice have definite "cleansing" qualities. Remaining on a fruit and vegetable juice diet for 3 to 5 days is not difficult, since there is no limitation to the quantity you may desire to drink. Drink as much pure water as you care to, and if distilled water is used, by adding a few drops of fresh lemon juice to each glassful the lost minerals are replaced. This could be considered a fast since no solid foods are eaten. When completing the

---

[1] The word "enema" refers to the injection of liquid into the rectum through the anus for the purpose of cleansing and evacuating the bowels. Many practitioners of the Mucusless Diet regularly use enemas and view it as a form of general hygiene. Ehret does not promote the use of unnatural laxative medications or store-bought saline enemas, such as a Fleet enemas. Many modern-day practitioners of the Mucusless Diet exclusively use lemon juice and distilled water enemas performed with a 2-quart enema bag, and not a bulb syringe. For detailed instructions about how to perform lemon enemas, see *Spira Speaks: Dialogs and Essays on the Mucusless Diet Healing System* by Prof. Spira.

experiment, make sure that the first meal is a "laxative" one. Ehret recommended sauerkraut (shredded cabbage) eaten with fresh celery stalks. Canned sauerkraut can be used by first draining off the liquid; add water and bring to a boil, then add one or two green pippin cooking apples, also a few dried prunes. Stew for at least an hour. The sauerkraut may be eaten either hot or cold. You should experience a bowel movement within 3 or 4 hours after eating. An evacuation before retiring is important, since poisons loosened during the juice fast should be completely eliminated as soon as possible. May we suggest that you reread Ehret's *Mucusless Diet* book, wherein he tells what is taking place during the cleansing diet and just what to expect. Do not retire before experiencing a "bowel movement" after breaking a fast, and an enema is recommended if necessary. The average individual does not properly digest an ordinary "meat meal" without putrefaction occurring. Needless to say, this poisonous putrefaction occurring in the digestive tract may develop such ailments as Bright's disease, pernicious anemia, goiter, scurvy and even tuberculosis. There is little doubt that human's health would be greatly improved if meat is left off the diet.

Note: Instead of canned sauerkraut, raw shredded cabbage is a cleaner alternative. For less mucused stomachs, a short fast may be broken with a meal of raw, mucusless fruits.

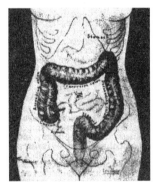

The Ideal Colon

The Large Bowel or Colon illustrated on the left is classically correct in its anatomical position and scale. Considerable variation occurs in the normal colon, depending on the type of individual.

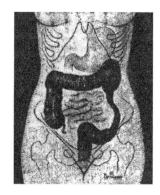

Spastic Constipation

Pinching down of the Descending Colon

Spastic constipation presents a history of flatulence and griping pains in the lower abdomen. Physicians have looked for this type in patients with a highly nervous temperament. The bowel muscles are pinched down and contraction waves are too severe.

The formation of our teeth and the length of our intestines prove that humans are not omnivorous, yet they follow the same omnivorous diet of the hog and other omnivorous animals. Willpower to resist the perverted habits to which we have become accustomed and the adoption of a frugivorous diet will bring about a recognizable regeneration in your physical and mental well-being within a few short months!

Of course, you know all about the harmful qualities of "cholesterol" and how our digestive organs find it impossible to properly dispose of any superfluous quantity. Cholesterol not only clogs the lining of the intestinal tract, but also can affect many of the vital organs of the body and cholesterol undoubtedly plays a considerable part in causing constipation. Every cook knows how grease and fats cling to the sidewalls of cooking utensils, especially pots and pans used in cooking meats. It is no easy matter to remove these fatty substances, and a lot of scouring is required. Yet, without giving it serious thought, the innocent cooks feed these harmful foods to their loved ones! Ample evidence exists proving the inability of the human digestive organs to digest or assimilate saturated fats and greases! The mistaken fallacy that meats are needed to supply necessary proteins to maintain a normal health balance makes it almost "sacrilegious" to oppose this belief. However, many physicians bravely admit that dairy products (milk, butter, cheese, and eggs) directly contribute to a large percentage of heart ailments because of their high cholesterol content.

Prof. Arnold Ehret considered all fatty foods as being harmful and extremely constipating—clogging up the intestinal tract, causing the entire system to become overloaded with their toxic waste. As we grow older, the body's vital energy is depleted; through faulty diet, elimination is practically stopped; the digestive organs are immobilized and unable to function—toxic, putrefactive wastes are retained; nerve energy is dissipated; and we become seriously ill. Improved habits of living, eating only non-constipating foods capable of "cleansing" the digestive tract (i.e., fresh fruits and starchless vegetables) become the proper procedure for regaining health. It is safe to say that 70 percent of the colons of the average person are impacted—some exceptionally so! "Grape sugar" (i.e. fruit sugar) is recognized as the energy-producing food element by many nutritionists, and all fruits and starchless vegetables are rich in this life-sustaining substance. The German chemist Ragnar Berg, in his book on *Food Chemistry*, classifies all vegetables and fruits as "alkaline," calling them "acid-binding," whereas grains and cereals (i.e., wheat, barley, oats, rice, and corn) as "acid-forming." In almost every instance, Chemist Berg's "acid-binding" foods are identical to those listed by Ehret as "mucusless" and Berg's "acid-forming" foods correspond with Ehret's "mucus-forming" foods. Chemist Berg found such dairy foods as eggs, butter, cheese, and "pasteurized milk" to be "acid-forming" and constipating. Many doctors recognize them as harmful because of their high "cholesterol" content. Prof. Ehret called them "mucus-forming."

Positive Healing Forces

We can only hope to attain the blessings of "Positive Healing Forces" through following proven health rules. Natural foods, physical exercises, deep breathing—PLUS a cheerful mental attitude! We human beings, in common with all other animals, possess the instinct of self-preservation. An inborn fear of losing our lives is strongly ingrained in our subconscious. It would seem unnecessary to tell what constipation is and what harm it does to the body, for no other ailment has been so thoroughly and consistently discussed. Constipation is the clogging up of the sewage system of the body!

The Need of Proteins

While we recognize proteins are essential in the human diet, we contend that Nature supplies sufficient proteins in natural fruits, starch-free vegetables, and nuts to fulfill our needs. Many physicians acknowledge this fact but their voices are completely drowned out by those who still consider meats, fish, and dairy products as a main source of protein. This conclusion may be traced to the fact that animal proteins leave very little residue. On the other side of the picture, we find that residue from fruits and vegetables is considerably more! This is just as nature would have it! The large bowel requires bulk before "mass action" or "evacuation" can take place. The residue from the decaying meat, fish, and dairy products, being insufficient to produce a bowel action, must first putrefy and is then absorbed by the circulation for elimination—while most of this poisonous waste remains in the bloodstream or is deposited in the tissues! The "bulk-residue" from fruits and vegetables are properly evacuated, since the main function of the large bowel is to rid the body of all waste products. If this process is turned over to the circulation, diseases that cause body wasting and resulting weakness can be expected to occur! Physics and purgatives cause constant irritation and overstimulating through constant use, which ultimately may prove injurious. While "regularity" must be observed, to do so through means of a violent purgative is often worse than the disease itself!

Foul breath, coated tongue, mental depression, loss of appetite, dull listless feeling, headaches, ringing in the ears, dizziness, skin eruptions, indigestion, belching, gas-bloat often accompanied by cramp-like pains, ulcers, and many kindred ailments are all the result of a long-standing constipation. Pimples, boils, and other skin injuries are directly brought about through Nature's use of the skin as a secondary eliminative organ:

Humans as "Scavengers"

Tracing human history back thousands of years, we find that they have *long* been a scavenger in their eating habits. They would voraciously stuff themselves with the dead carcass of birds and animals that they had learned to slaughter even in their primitive stage. Not knowing where or when their next meal was coming from, they would gorge themselves on the food available. Their life in Paradise ended when they changed from their fruitarian existence to meat eating! They have turned their intestinal tract into a "burial place" for putrefying, decaying animal foods. With the recent innovation of chemical "retardants" used to prevent "spoliation" in preserved foods, both bottled and canned, these chemical additives increase their "shelf life." Even green vegetables are grown for acceptance in the marketplace rather than their nutritional value! The search for greater financial profits supersedes consideration of food values! We pasteurize, homogenize, dehydrate, adulterate, emulsify, and devitalize our food with cheap fillers, coal-tar dyes, chemical bleaches, "US certified" artificial coloring—whatever that might mean—and even "formaldehyde," which everyone knows as an embalming fluid! Our leading manufacturers use "half truths" in their advertising, and very often even outright lies are told in advertising many of today's leading food products. And we accept these food substitutes as "pure, wholesome food." Take time to read the label on the next loaf of bread you buy—or any of the bakery products for that matter! The Pure Food Laws require listing of all artificial ingredients—yet the use of "artificial flavors," "propyl paraben," and other chemicals used to retard "spoliation" is legal. The effect these "retardants" have on delicate mucus membrane and the lining of our intestinal tract has not as yet been divulged—but you may be sure that they play an important part in the cause of constipation. Next time you are shopping—"pass up" the enticingly illustrated frozen "TV dinners" and the patented "moist" cake recipes "so easy to prepare!" Stop cheating your body of the essential life giving foods. Every mouthful of fried, greasy food is a mouthful too much! Failure to pay proper attention to the desire for a bowel movement or to devote sufficient time to it, leads to a retarded movement and later to constipation. Every individual living today is faced with the possibility of suffering either mental or physical breakdown, or both, through some expected, disabling, painful disease! These almost certain results are directly attributable to present-day living—surely not an especially pleasing outlook! Increasing evidence has been found that habitual environmental distress, repressed anxiety, grief, envy, hate, fear, worry, and frustrations of all kinds cause constipation and often result in physical breakdown through organic changes.

Foodless Foods

A great majority of the people residing in the United States were raised on refined white flour products, refined and imitation sugars, artificial flavoring, and coloring extracts, all of which are unnatural foods totally unacceptable by the human body. The discovery through illness in later life that only natural foods are intended for the human body seems to come as a distinct "shock," and total acceptance is not an easy matter. Adapting natural living methods will bring worthwhile results, and this great boon of health and happiness is within your reach; grasp it firmly and hold tightly! Civilization, with all of its perverse habits has brought about the present decadence of mankind, proving conclusively the complete inability of the human body to adjust to an artificial, sophisticated manner of living. Only through living in harmony with Nature's teachings can these destructive disorders be corrected. Fresh fruits and vegetables remain generally undesirable to the average individual, through hidden fear of possible harmful results! The teachings of Arnold Ehret have brought about an understanding of why and how the very foods actually "cleansing" the bloodstream were wrongly condemned, tabooed, and discontinued! Through the teachings of this great benefactor of humanity, untold thousands now know the blessing of joyous "good health." Dr. J. H. Kellogg of Battle Creek fame wrote, "Our health is made or unmade at the table! Your natural appetite will demand the foods your body requires, and it will be found that the easiest way is to consume food in its natural state. Whenever we eat "wrong foods"—even though but once a month— *our* dormant diseased cells grasp the opportunity to resuscitate themselves, and only through total abstinence from these "wrong foods" can you expect to completely free yourself from illness."

Arnold Ehret's *Mucusless Diet Healing System* teaches that "constipation is a clogging up of the entire human pipe-system. Nature wisely stores the undigested, toxic wastes "temporarily" in the tissues, awaiting an early opportunity to dispose of these poisons! Sickness is such an opportunity—acute disease is Nature's attempt to eliminate the stored-up 'sewage' and the 'healing process' differs according to the physical condition of each individual." Most emphatically—we cannot afford to ignore constipation as a minor ailment! The very secret of Vitality lies in the ability of the body to eliminate these waste materials clogging the tissues and the intestinal tract. It is your duty to aid Nature's efforts through eating natural foods to keep yourself free from disease!

More Causes of Constipation

Eating a large breakfast of indigestible proteins, such as "hot cakes," waffles, French toast, oatmeal, bacon, and eggs—washed down with a large cup of hot coffee; rushing to work immediately upon rising— often with insufficient sleep—makes it practically impossible for the digestive organs to function at all. And the final result is a deep-rooted constipated condition! Add to all this the combination of sedentary habits, plus a "one-sided" heavy starch, "bread, meat, and mashed potato" diet. Constipation, being basic to every disease known to humankind from the simple cold to pneumonia—makes it difficult to understand how the average individual still believes in a "cure" merely through taking a "four-way pill," an "anti-cold" tablet, or some "patent" medicine. We quote from a recent newspaper article:

> Millions of Americans falsely assume that there are easy ways to stay well and youthful looking, and resist the necessary arduous and disciplinary requirements of really caring for the complex, finely tuned, vulnerable body each of us inherits. Instead they turn, among other things, to diet fads, patent medicines, a countless variety of pills, and inadequate exercise. Our affluence has reduced physical exertion and increased "overeating," excess drinking, smoking, late hours and drug consumption. A false sense of well-being leads many people to assume that illness cannot strike them, or that cures are to be taken for granted, laboring under the illusion that "miracles of medicine will keep them well"! —*Anonymous doctor*

We thank you, Doctor, for you most excellent summation of the facts.

The Simplest Meals Are BEST!

Starting with today—instead of your customary meal of "meat, bread, and mashed potatoes," try eating a crisp, fresh green-leaf salad using grated carrots and chopped celery, plus the addition or one or two cooked vegetables (such as peas, or string beans, squash, or beets, etc.) with a few slices of fresh tomatoes added. If bread is used, it should be thoroughly toasted and eaten dry. Avoid drinking liquids of any kind with meals. If your preference is for fresh, tree-ripened fruit make the entire meal consist of crisp lettuce leaves and the fruits you desire. All fruits blend harmoniously. No starches (i.e., bread or cakes) should be eaten with fruit salad. After a few days of this type of food, you will be delighted to note that worthwhile results are already being experienced! Unless you are actually hungry—DON'T eat! Dr. Jonathan Formam, MD, English physician, writes, "If we were to use the knowledge regarding foods that is now available to us, sickness could be wiped out in one generation!"

You should by now be fully conversant with the life-giving foods meant for human consumption; foods that are best for you—fit to eat—foods that produce good health, strength, and vitality! But we cannot stress too frequently the dangers of overeating—of even the best foods. There is much more danger in eating too much than of eating too little! AVOID OVEREATING!

Retain Good Health Indefinitely
We have always maintained that the condition known as "constipation" is a direct invitation for disease! The individual is deliberately seeking illness—just so long as he or she permits constipation to exist. There is only one disease, although it has various manifestations. There is only one cause—waste-toxic matters retained in the system! During every moment of life, waste is being formed by the destruction of tissue, and this waste must be promptly removed to insure good health! You will find it necessary to call upon your Willpower and Determination to follow through and overcome Constipation—but you will find the reward well worth the effort.

Eating natural foods will bring improvement in both your physical and mental health. You may expect to experience slight abdominal pains occasionally and possible "gassy bloating" accompanied by belching. Should the pains become annoying, try drinking a full glass of pure, warm or hot water. If the pains continue, discontinue all fresh fruits restricting your diet to cooked vegetables only—until the pains have subsided, before returning to the fruit diet. The aggressive elimination of the fresh fruits stirs up poisons, while cooked vegetables are much less "aggressive" in their cleansing ability.

37

> Whatsoever Nature expels is waste and foreign matter. When the body is overloaded with encumbrances—plainly the result of decomposing, indigestible, retained foods—these morbid matters must be eliminated, or loss of health through auto-intoxication will inevitably result. —*Prof. Arnold Ehret*

When normal bowel functioning is insufficient, Nature resorts to other methods of elimination—i.e., boils, carbuncles, ulcers, and abscess—to name but a few. All of which definitely signifies that the body is desperately striving to eliminate this unwanted surplus. The commonly accepted belief is that these foods must be replaced—and the sufferer is incorrectly advised to increase the daily intake rather than decrease! Recognition of the truth takes place when the patient is practically at death's point. This terrible "tragedy of errors" occurs until we finally arrive at a full realization that "Nature's laws cannot be ignored." We must no longer permit ourselves to remain unimpressed with Nature healing abilities! Normal health depends upon correction of "our" misleading errors. There are, to course, many factors that can cause constipation. An abnormally slow movement of fecal matter through the large intestine is most always associated with a large amount of dry, hard feces in the descending colon. This condition results through neglect or failure to respond immediately to the defecation urge; in fact, quite often withheld and not permitted to occur. The prolonged use of mineral oils has been known to bring about severe constipation, as do many of the commonly used constipation remedies. Both prescription as well as nonprescription drugs, including headache tablets, antihistamines, aspirin, sleeping pills, muscle relaxants, opiates, narcotics, and tranquilizers are recognized contributors and must be avoided! Practically everyone today is to a greater or lesser extent encumbered with latent, morbid matter which in itself represents a constipated condition, and the medical name given the illness merely identifies the particular part of the body or organ where the illness exists! Our bloodstream supplies nourishment to every part of the body and only through fallowing Nature's biological law and eating proper foods as provided by Nature can we ensure our bodies a clean, vital bloodstream. Natural health teachings are presumably techniques followed only by "food faddists" and "health cranks," and it is high time the unfortunate sick and ailing individuals exchange their "blind faith" in the "surgeon's scalpel" and dependency of medical drugs in the hope of overcoming their ailments—for the aid that Nature offers! The versatility and magnitude of natural healing has been conclusively proven over the years—even though medical science has as yet failed to arrive at a willingness to accept these basic facts.

In Conclusion

Our colon is the seat of all disease and therefore the preservation and restoration of health is solely dependent upon Internal Cleanliness! Life itself consists of a continual process of tearing down and building anew.

The average individual carries around as much as 10 pounds of uneliminated feces. Continually carrying this mass of filth, day after day during his or her entire life, re-absorbing its poisons back into the circulation, is surely a detriment to health. The engorged intestines, reeking with filth and putrefaction, poison the bloodstream, which feeds every vital organ. These poisons are steadily being re-absorbed into the circulation while in a semi-liquid state. A constant circulation takes place between the fluid content of the bowel causing every portion of this poisonous blood to pass several times during 24-hour period into the alimentary canal. The so-called "daily bowel movement" is no assurance that the individual is not the victim of costiveness, since the age-old, solid encrustations clinging to the intestinal wall permit passage of fecal matter through a small aperture of the intestines permitting daily bowel functioning to take place. An unnatural distension of the colon to several times its normal size results; and this impacted colon is a veritable hotbed for breeding disease germs and poisonous toxins. An exclusive diet of natural foods—fruits and starchless vegetables—purifies and cleanses the colon!

Health is an inestimable blessing never fully appreciated until it has slipped from our grasp! Perfect health is the spice of life, and may those who enjoy this blessing retain it indefinitely! May *those* who have *lost* it regain it soon, so that they may realize the joy of living! Nothing worthwhile comes easily!

Nature alone heals all ailments, and only through complete acceptance of Nature's teachings can the survival of civilization be assured. FAITH, PERSEVERANCE, PERSISTENCE, and

WILLPOWER contain the necessary ingredients to bring about GOOD health and the ability to OVERCOME CONSTIPATION NATURALLY.

"The journey of a thousand miles starts with but a single step!" (Chinese proverb)—We wish you "Godspeed" on your journey to better health!

FINIS

List of Other Publications

PROF. ARNOLD EHRET'S
MUCUSLESS DIET HEALING SYSTEM
ANNOTATED, REVISED, AND EDITED BY PROF. SPIRA

After almost 100 years, the *Mucusless Diet Healing System* has been revised and annotated for twenty-first-century audiences!

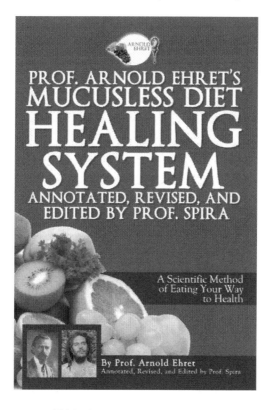

This is a must-read for all people interested in the Mucusless Diet!

Find it at www.mucusfreelife.com/revised-mucusless-diet

41

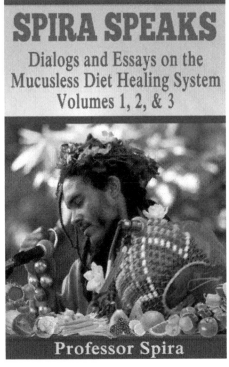

Join Prof. Spira for an unprecedented look into the healing power of a mucus-free lifestyle! After losing 110 pounds and overcoming numerous physical ailments, Spira learned that he had a gift for articulating the principles of the diet through writing and music. As he began to interact with health-seekers on the internet in 2005, he realized that written dialogs about the diet could benefit far more than just its intended readers. This book is a compilation of the best writings by Professor Spira on the subject.

What is the *Mucusless Diet Healing System*? How has it helped numerous people overcome illnesses thought to be permanent? What does it take to practice a mucus-free lifestyle in the twenty-first century? Why is the transition diet one of the most misunderstood aspects of the mucusless diet? Spira answers these questions and much more in his unprecedented new eBook that contains never-before released writings about the mucusless diet.

Visit www.mucusfreelife.com/spira-speaks

Prof. Arnold Ehret's Rational Fasting for Physical, Mental, and Spiritual Rejuvenation: Introduced and Edited by Prof. Spira

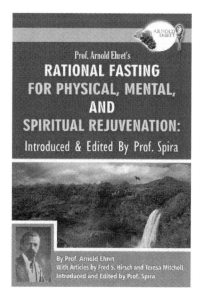

Discover one of Ehret's most vital and influential works, and companion the the Mucusless Diet Healing System. Introducing *Rational Fasting for Physical, Mental, and Spiritual Rejuvenation: Introduced and Edited by Prof. Spira*, now available from Breathair Publishing.

In this masterpiece, Ehret explains how to successfully, safely, and rationally conduct a fast in order to eliminate harmful waste from the body and promote internal healing. Also included are famous essays on Ehret's teachings by Fred Hirsch and long-time devotee Teresa Mitchell.

You will learn:

- The Common Fundamental Cause in the Nature of Diseases
- Complete Instructions for Fasting
- Building a Perfect Body through Fasting
- Important Rules for the Faster
- How Long to Fast
- Why to Fast
- When and How to Fast
- How Teresa Mitchell Transformed Her Life through Fasting
- And Much More!

43

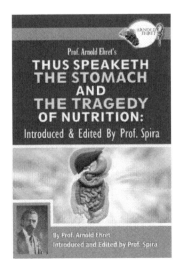 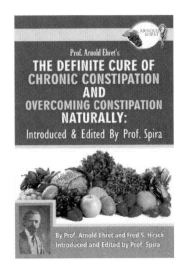

Thus Speaketh the Stomach and A Tragedy of Nutrition

If your intestines could talk, what would they say? What if you could understand health through the perspective of your stomach? In this unprecedented work, Arnold Ehret gives voice to the stomach and reveals the foundation of human illness.

The Definite Cure of Chronic Constipation and Overcoming Constipation Naturally: Introduction by Prof. Spira

In the Definite Cure of Chronic Constipation and Overcoming Constipation Naturally, Prof. Arnold Ehret and his number-one student Fred Hirsch explore generally constipated condition of the human organism.

COMING SOON!!!

The Art of Transition: Spira's *Mucusless Diet Healing System* Menu and Recipe Guide

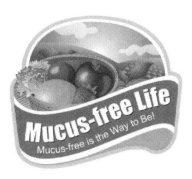

What does a mucusless diet practitioner actually eat? What kind of transitional mucus-forming foods are best? What are the most effective menu combinations to achieve long-lasting success with the mucusless diet? What are the best transitional cooked and raw menus? What foods and combinations should be avoided at all costs? How can you prepare satisfying mucusless and mucus-lean meals for your family?

These questions and much more will be addressed in Prof. Spira's long-awaited mucusless diet menu and recipe eBook! Stay tuned!

Introduction

Purpose

Popular Fruits, Vegetables, and Vegan Items Omitted from this Book

Organic vs. Non-organic

    Mucus-lean

    Raw vs. Cooked

    Satisfying Nut and Dried Fruit Combinations

The Onion Sauté

Filling Steamed and Baked Vegetable Meals

Spira's Special "Meat-Away" Meal

Mucusless

Raw Combination Salads

Raw Dressings

Favorite Mono-fruit Meals

Favorite Dried Fruits

Favorite Fruit Combinations

Vegetable Juices

Fruit Smoothies and Sauces

Fresh Fruit Juices

Sample Combinations and Weekly Menus

Projected Release: Winter 2014

SPIRA'S MUCUSLESS DIET
COACHING & CONSULTATIONS

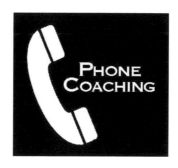

After receiving a consultation with Professor Spira, I was able to take my practice of the Mucusless Diet Healing System to a new level. Speaking face to face with an advanced practitioner was key and a true blessing on my journey. I'm looking forward to following up with another in the future!

-Brian Stern, Certified Bikram Yoga Instructor and Musician

You truly are amazing. You have done nothing but given all you can to help me and I truly appreciate this. Thank you for "feeding me."

-Samantha Claire, Pianist and Educator

Spira has practiced the mucusless diet and studied the natural hygienic/back-to-nature movements for the past 10 years. During that time, he has advised and helped many in the art of transitioning away from mucus-forming foods. For a limited time, talk with Prof. Spira about your individual needs, challenges, and questions. Skype, telephone, or in-person consultations available! For more information, visit:

www.mucusfreelife.com/diet-coaching

Visit the MUCUSFREELIFE.COM Amazon store for great deals on

Arnold Ehret's Classic Writings

WEB LINKS

Websites

mucusfreelife.com

breathairmusic.com

Facebook

Prof. Spira Fan Page: www.facebook.com/ProfessorSpira

Arnold Ehret Fan Page: www.facebook.com/arnoldehret.us

Arnold Ehret Support Group: www.facebook.com/groups/arnoldehret/

YouTube

Prof. Spira's Breathair-Vision: www.youtube.com/user/professorspira

Twitter

@profspira

@ArnoldEhret1

Visit our Bookstore to Find Books by Arnold Ehret!

www.mucusfreelife.com/storefront/

Spira is now available for mucusless diet consultations/coaching!

www.mucusfreelife.com/storefront/product/mucusless-diet-coaching/

Please Share Your Reviews!

Share your reviews and comments about this book and your experiences with the mucusless diet on Amazon and mucusfreelife.com. Prof. Spira would love to hear how the text has helped you.

PEACE, LOVE, AND BREATH!

Printed in Great Britain
by Amazon

54666574R00034